Message from Author

Having once been overweight myself, I can very well relate to people who have issues with their body. I made a major transition from a heavy junk food consumer to a healthy person and I can tell you, it's no joke. When I first decided to start a healthy lifestyle, I found myself exposed to a huge amount of information, way too huge. I was bombarded by infomercials of DVD workouts,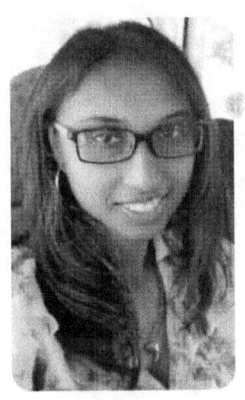

diets, etc. I had a really hard time making choices. However, I have now achieved my ideal weight and I can proudly say that I have a fit and toned body, my dream body. Unfortunately, I have to admit, this should have occurred a long time back. It would, if only I didn't spend so much time in the jungle of information out there. This is the reason why I am now writing my own health and fitness books; precise and informative. You'll get the exact information you want without the pain of filtering out what's truly relevant and what's not. And I can guarantee you that my recommendations will bring the results you're looking for.

Miss B. Rawiyah Mulung,

Fitness Coach,

Blogger,

Writer

I0450551

This book is dedicated to all the people out there who feel they will never achieve their dream body. "You only truly fail when you stop trying".

DIET TIPS

1) **A small plate is always better than a larger one.** To avoid overeating, you may prefer to use a small plate rather than a larger one. When you place a certain amount of food on your plate, it can either look significantly little or it may seem to be just enough. For instance, imagine placing an amount of food on a large plate. The empty space all around can really get to you and you may get trapped in the psychological reaction that you need more food. However, if you use a small plate with the same amount of food taking up all the space on your plate, you'll automatically feel that you are consuming enough food. You avoid significant overeating.

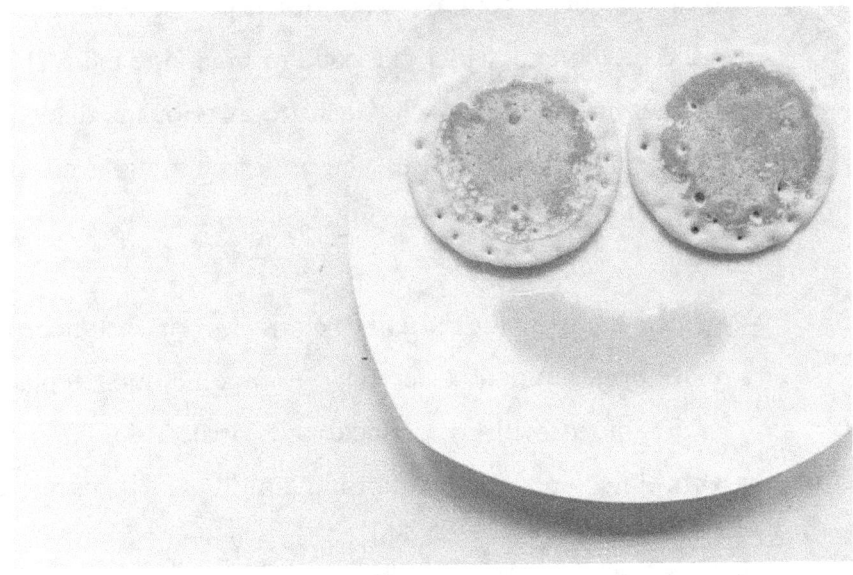

2) **Avoid the bad carbs.** These are the ones to be held responsible for that stubborn belly fat. Be cautious here. Only avoid the bad carbs, not the good ones. Wholegrain is still okay to consume. To be on the safe side, I only stick to eating a carb filled food once a day. For example, I usually eat a slice of wholegrain bread for breakfast. The only other way I consume carbs throughout the rest of the day is through vegetables. These are the good carbs.

3) **Try using an online calories counter**. There are many websites out there which provide you with the calorie count option. You might be thinking that you do not need this or that you can already estimate your amount of calories, but let me tell you that you will be surprised once you start using the online calories counter. Very often, people tend to overlook little ingredients which they add or misjudge the real amount of food in their plate. This leads to a serious underestimation of the amount of calories you are consuming. And then you wonder why you not losing those extra pounds.

4) **Make healthy ingredients' choices.** For instance, replace that normal tomato sauce with an organic one. Replace your white bread with wholemeal one. Instead of eating those chocolate cereals in the morning, opt for a wholegrain cereal. Choose cereals with blueberries which are a belly fat reducing food. There's a huge variety of healthy products out there. You just need to reach out to them.

5) **Choose the right snacks.** Snacking is inevitable. It's not always about whether we are hungry or not, sometimes snacking time is just a way to relax or socialise. You might think that a little snack from time to time is nothing significant. However, bad snacks could be doing more bad to your waistline than you think. If the first thing you grab when it's snacking time is one chocolate cookie, you are on the wrong track. You could be munching on nuts at that time. Almonds, for instance, make great snacks and fill you up.

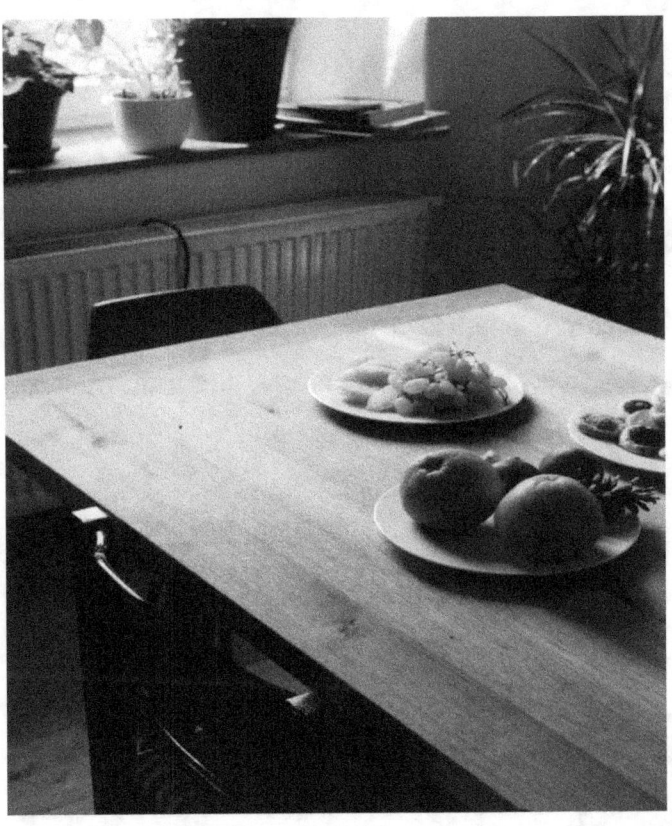

6) **Tailor your pre-workout and post-workout meals as per your workout.** You make a huge mistake by skipping on those pre-workout and especially post-workout meals. These meals are meant to fuel you up for your exercises and to help your muscles recover after workout. You should, of course, tailor these meals according to the type of exercise you indulge in. For instance, 20 minutes High Intensity Interval Training will clearly require much more fuelling than a 20 minutes jog.

7) **Drink a lot of water.** This is one typical line that you must have heard endless times in your life. However, drinking water could play a major role in aiding your weight loss. Besides the numerous health benefits which water has to offer, it also acts as an appetite suppressant. It is recommended to drink water both before and after a meal. The reason for this is because the water makes you feel full. It prevents you from overeating.

8) **Never skip breakfast.** Research has shown that people who take breakfast on a daily basis attain a much higher weight loss level than people who skip breakfast. During sleeping hours, our body goes into an inactive mode causing our metabolism to slow down significantly. Breakfast on the other hand, boosts the metabolism and also prevents us from over-eating at lunch time or from snacking too often throughout the day.

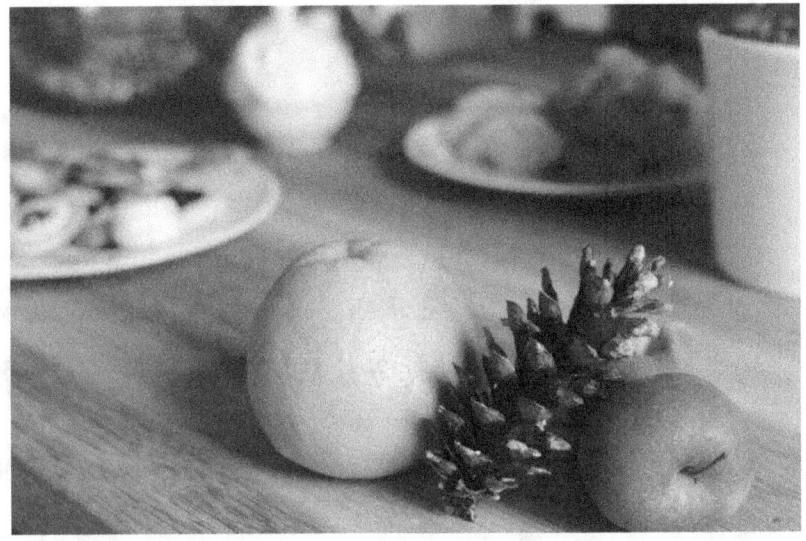

9) **Have the right breakfast.** Your breakfast may not contain enough protein. Ideally, breakfast should be a low-carb, high-protein one. According to a research published in the International Journal of Obesity, participants who ate a protein-packed breakfast consumed 26 percent fewer calories at lunch than those who ate a calorically identical meal with less protein.

10) **Eat a lot of Blueberries.** Not only are these tasty and juicy, but they work wonders for your belly fat. This is particularly appealing to many of us because we all know that no matter how much weight we lose, the belly fat is always the most stubborn one which doesn't seem to move an inch! But what is in blueberries that seems to work magic? It is actually just

the antioxidants found in these marvellously juicy little things.

11) **Opt for Olive Oil.** When it comes to healthy dieting, olive oil might be just what you need. It tastes great, contains good-for-your-heart healthy fats and helps you lose unwanted belly fat. Olive oil is rich in monounsaturated fatty acids (MUFA). Research indicates that replacing other types of fats with monounsaturated fats, especially olive oil, helps people lose weight without additional food restriction or physical activity.

12) **Avoid emotional eating at all costs.** Our first reaction to stress or emotional pressure is usually grabbing a chocolate cake or a cookie or simply overeating. It is not the solution. You should find healthy ways to calm yourself. You could try yoga, exercise, taking a walk or soaking in a hot bath. If you're lonely or bored, reach out to others instead of reaching out for the food. Call a friend, socialise. You'll feel better.

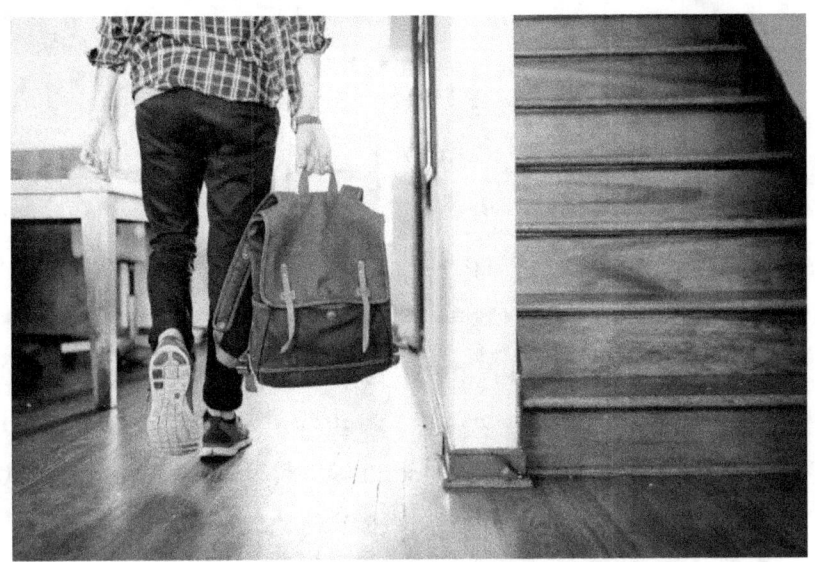

13) **Eating fewer calories does not mean eating less food.** This is a popular misconception that people have. You can fill up while on a diet, as long as you choose your foods wisely. Enjoy whole fruits, leafy salads, and green veggies of all kinds. Select beans of any kind. Add them to soups, salads, and entrees, or enjoy them as a hearty dish on their own. Try high-fiber cereal, oatmeal, brown rice, whole-wheat pasta, whole-wheat or multigrain bread.

14) **You will not lose weight faster if you eat less.** If you eat too few calories per day, your body could enter into a starvation mode. Your metabolism will actually slow down and slow your ability to lose weight. In general, women should not go below 1,200 calories and men shouldn't go below 1,500 calories.

15) **Get enough sleep.** The connection between sleep and weight loss may not seem very clear to you. However, sleep deprivation causes weight gain. Research has shown that people who sleep less tend to eat more. They find it necessary to have snacks to boost their energy throughout the day. These people are also less apt to exercise. They just do not feel up for it because of their low energy level from sleep deprivation. Lack of sleep also slows down your metabolism. That is, you burn fewer calories than you would if you had slept enough.

16) **Make smoothies your best friend.** Healthy, convenient and portable, smoothies are ideal fuel-on-the-go for breakfast, an afternoon snack or dessert. Smoothies provide important protein, vitamins and minerals. Smoothies also make great pre-workout as well as post-workout meals.

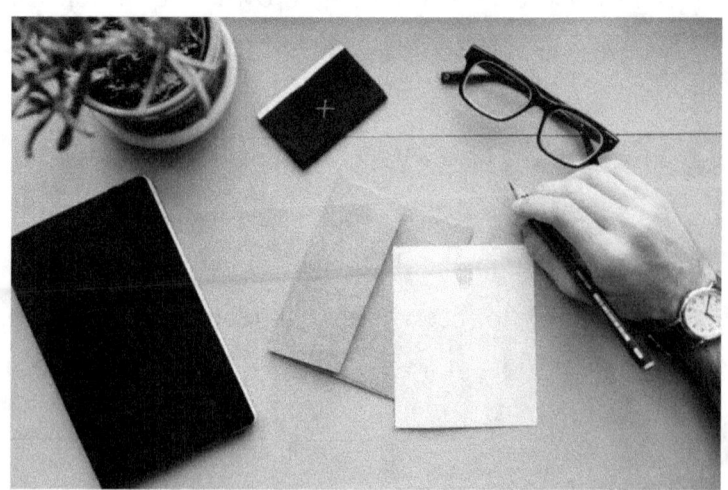

17) **Make a list before hitting the grocery stores.** This is very important if you do not want to end up with three bars of chocolate, one packet of six cookies, two litres of fizzy drinks or with a fast-food! Only include healthy items in your list. If you're unsure whether a foodstuff is healthy or not, find information on the Internet about that product. It will save you the trouble of wondering about it while shopping.

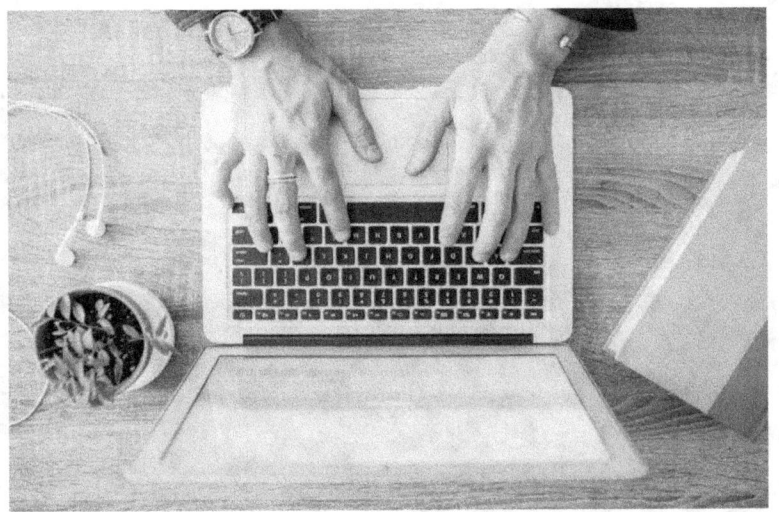

18) **Ensure that your grocery store list is only made up of healthy items.** This can be particularly difficult if you have the habit of sticking to certain products or brands. Again, surf the Internet. There's a world of information waiting for you out there. Find healthy alternatives to the products you usually buy. Read customer reviews. You might end up with something even better than you thought.

19) **Read the labels.** Food product labels can be very confusing. However, there are a few tips to follow if you're on a weight loss journey. Watch out for the calories. The higher the amount of calories, the more damaging it is for your body. Pay attention to the amount of carbs, proteins and fibre most essentially. A healthy combination would be low carb-high protein-high fibre.

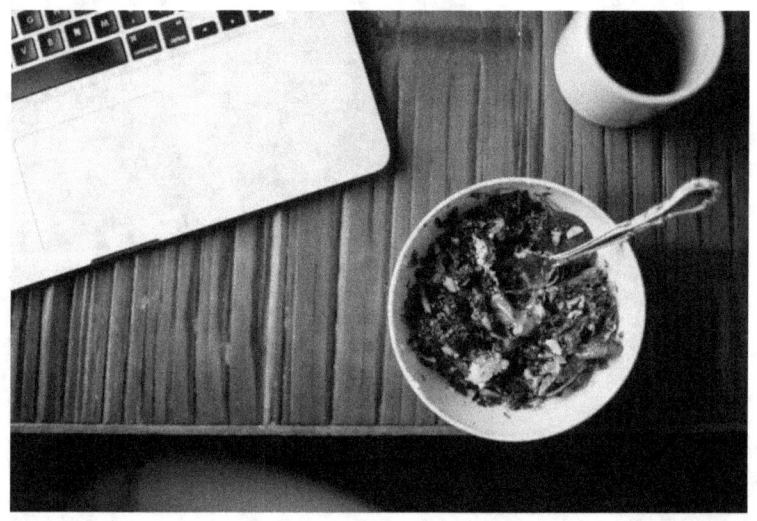

20) **Boost your fibre intake.** With fiber filled foods, you get to eat more with fewer calories. This is because high-fibre diets tend to be less energy dense. Also, fibre requires more chewing time. This allows your body to register when you're full and it prevents you from overeating. High-fibre diets also give the impression that the diet is larger and you therefore feel fuller for a longer time.

FITNESS TIPS

21) **Go for compound exercises.** These are full body exercises working multiple muscle groups at the same time. Obviously, they prove to be one of the most effective types of exercises you can possible do. Compound exercises include squats, lunges, bench press, pull-ups, deadlifts and many more.

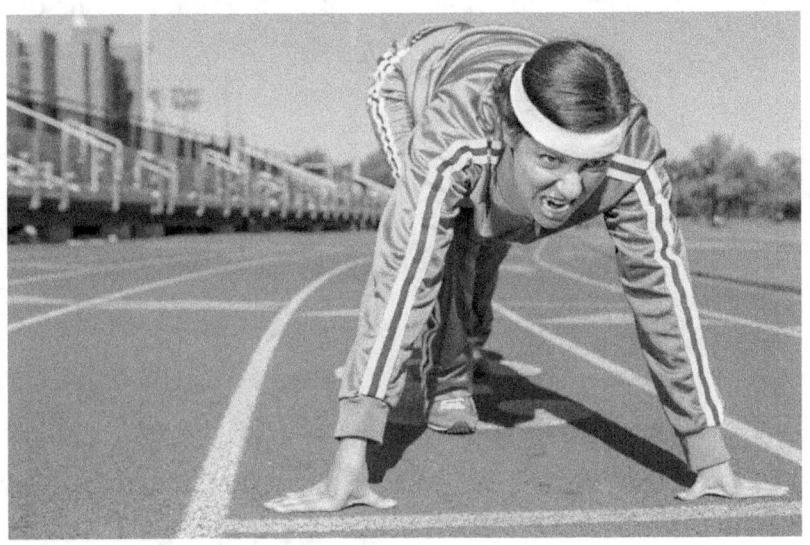

22) **Choose High Intensity Interval Training.** Often referred to as HIIT, this is a very intense type of training. You make your heart rate shoot up for a certain time interval and take an active recovery for another and start again. Your heart rate gets the chance to lower down during the active recovery period. Interval training allows you to exercise at higher

intensities for a much longer period of time than steady state, so you burn more fat.

23) **Always warm-up before exercise.** The purpose of warming up is to prepare the body for the conditioning or stimulus of the exercise session by increasing blood flow to the heart and to the exercising muscles, which serves to warm up and loosen up muscles. Warm-up activities should undeniably be an essential part of any exercise program. It is one of the best ways to avoid any injury.

24) **Always cool-down and stretch after a workout.** Cooling down will return the body to pre-exercise conditions and reduce muscle soreness. Take the time to lower your heart rate by cooling down for about five minutes, and then perform stretches. Stretching improves flexibility, helps to disperse lactic acid that can build up during the exercise session and helps to prepare the body for the next workout.

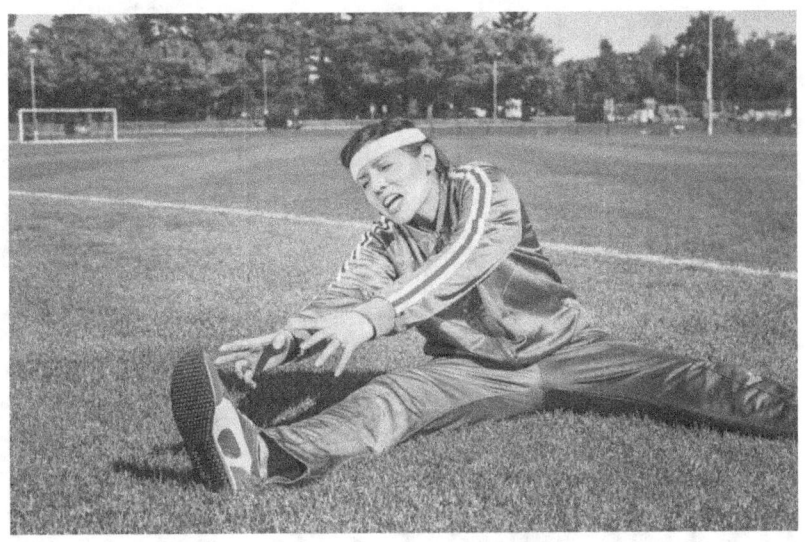

25) **Do dynamic warm-up exercises.** A dynamic warm-up uses stretches that are "dynamic," meaning you are moving as you stretch. Dynamic stretching is ideal as the core of a warm-up routine. It activates muscles you will use during your workout. Dynamic stretching improves range of motion and improves body awareness. Warming up in motion enhances muscular performance and power.

26) **Do more squats.** Squatting has more benefits than you think, both for men and women. Being a compound, full-body exercise, squats work multiple muscles in your body at the same time. Squats also burn more calories per rep than almost any other move! They boost your performance by making you jump higher and run faster. Also, squats work your glutes to a large extent.

27) **Take up a fitness trainer's job.** If you have reached an advanced level of fitness and you do not suffer from any medical conditions, you might consider making a living from your passion for fitness. Fitness trainers are very popular nowadays. They can almost be ranked as famous as some celebrities. Successful and professional fitness trainers earn a considerable amount of money and get the fame as the bonus.

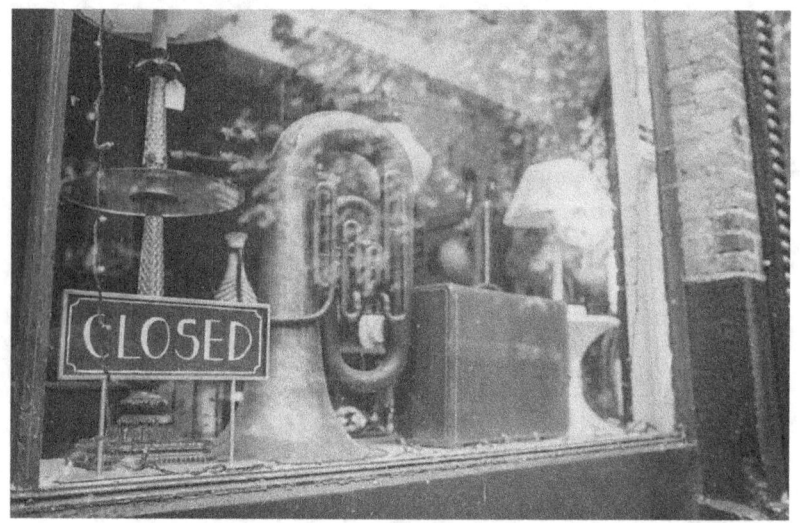

28) **Get rid of the thought that there's a fixed time to exercise.** The plain truth is that any time is a good time to exercise. Some people stick to morning workouts for months and when they suddenly have some other priority in the morning, they completely miss out on the workout. It doesn't have to be that way. Be it 6am, 4pm or even 10pm, if you haven't yet done your workout for the day, just get it done.

29) **Consider DVD workouts.** When you follow a DVD workout, you tend to be more committed and more attentive to your workout than when you are on your own at the gym. The fitness trainer in the DVD will be instructing you and encouraging you throughout the workout. You'll be exercising alongside other people in the DVD. And you won't end up taking unnecessary breaks.

30) **Be active whenever you can.** For example, you could be taking a stroll while talking on the phone instead of just lying in the couch and talking. Standing burns more calories than sitting which in turn burns more calories than lying down. Use this information. Instead of sitting in your office chair, stand up and type. Some offices have in-built features where the computer screens can be moved to a higher level to allow employees to stand up and work when they wish to do so.

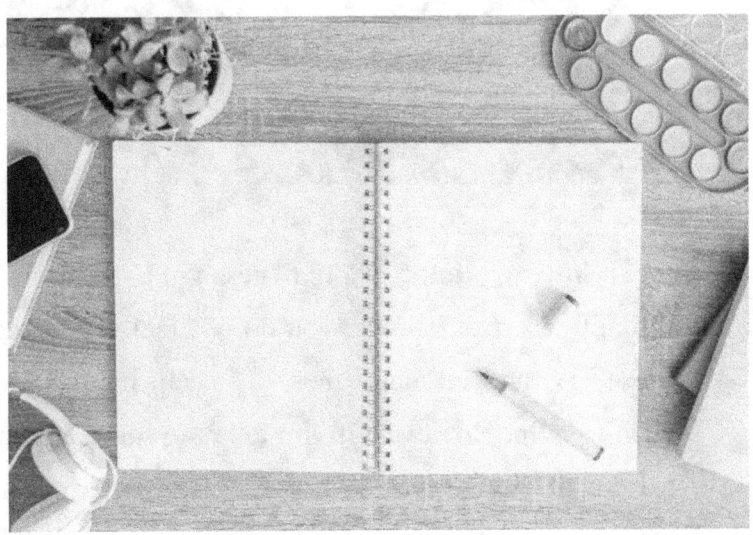

31) **Set yourself a fitness goal.** This goal can be anything you wish. It can be losing extra pounds, getting a flat belly, getting a toned body, etc... Setting a goal before you start a workout routine is important to keep you on track. Whenever you do not feel like exercising, remind yourself of that goal and of what you'll be losing on if you do not exercise. It will help you push yourself and get things done. Stick to having one goal at a time otherwise you'll only be inviting disappointment in.

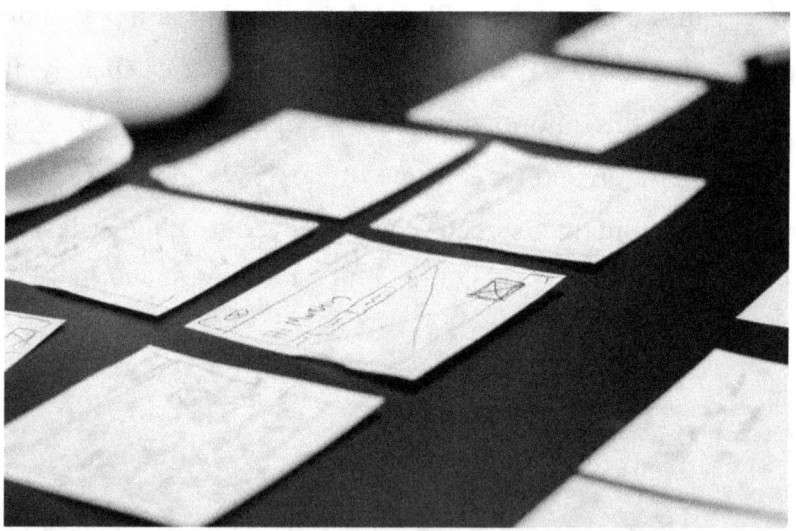

32) **Learn how to stick to your fitness goal.** This can be a very difficult task. Sometimes, you do not feel motivated enough to exercise and in such times, a goal in mind might not do much to help. However, if you take the same goal and put it in front of your eyes, it will have a greater impact on you. For instance, stick up your fitness role model's picture in

your room. Whenever you look at that picture, you'll be reminded of what you can and will achieve.

33) **Take a day off.** It is essential that you take a rest day when you're on a workout program. It is usually recommended that you take one rest day every week or two days off per week if the workout is very intense. This rest day is very much required for your muscles and your body to recuperate. Pushing yourself and not taking that day off will only lead to a decreased performance in the following workout days. It might even be cause for injury.

34) **Change your exercise environment.** Sometimes, we get bored at the very idea of going to the same old gym every single day. This is why you should change your exercise environment once in a while. For example, you could jog on the beach and still get your workout done. You can show up at a friend who has a home gym and ask to workout in his gym for a day. You can go hiking for a change.

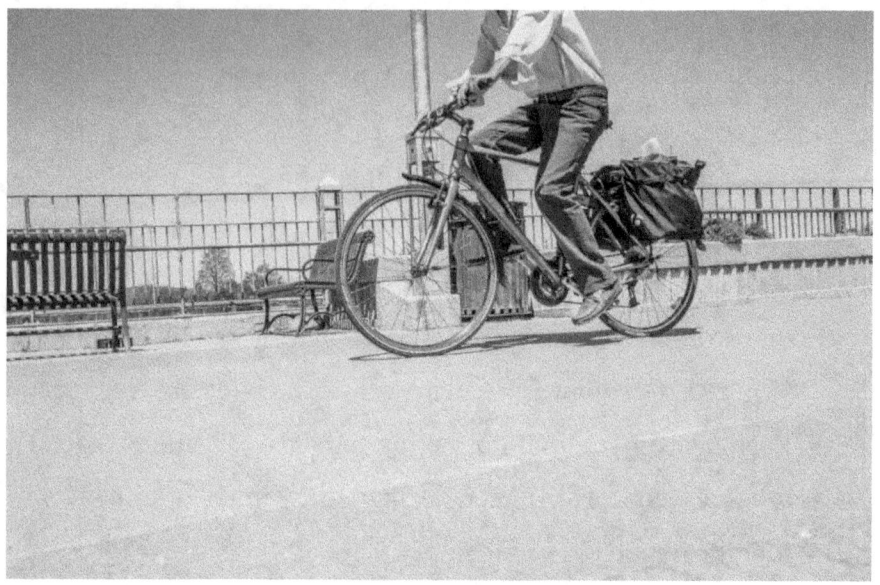

35) **Make exercising interesting.** Doing the same exercise routine all over can get boring with time. There are hundreds of different types of exercises out there from which you can choose and mix up. Incorporate new moves or modifications in your workout routine every now and then and you'll find that it gets less boring when you're always trying out something new. You'll even look forward to exercise time.

36) **Get motivated.** It is highly important that you stay motivated when you are on your fitness journey. You can do so by joining fitness groups. These are usually groups on social media which comprise of fitness lovers. They encourage and support each other. Or you can simply get inspired by downloading fitness quotes and sticking them around the house. These are pretty motivational.

37) **Have a workout buddy.** When you follow the same fitness routine and exercise with a friend, you feel more accountable. You feel the obligation to stay on track. The same goes for your friend. In this way, you make sure both of you stay on the right track. Motivation is also higher when you exercise with your fitness buddy. You get to encourage each other. It goes without saying that, in trying to motivate others, we often end up motivating ourselves.

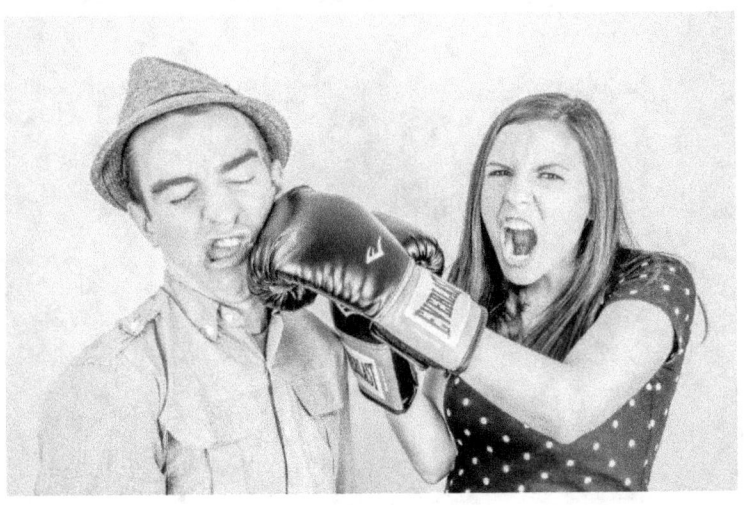

If you like this book, make sure to check out my other fitness and health books:

"Compound exercises: Exercise The Right Way" –
By B.Rawiyah Mulung

Available on Amazon stores and
in e-book version on Amazon Kindle Store.
Or buy it from createspace.com (an Amazon company) at
https://www.createspace.com/5241058?ref=1147694&utm_id=6026

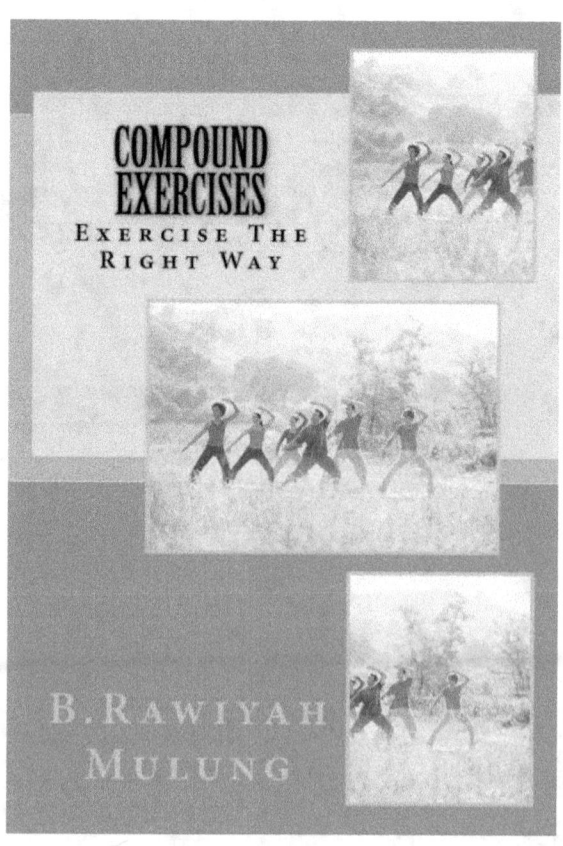

Also, subscribe to my blog at

http://yourfitnesshealth.blogspot.com

Or, follow my facebook page at

http://www.facebook.com/yourfitnesshealthblog

I'll always bring to you the best in the field

of fitness and health ☺

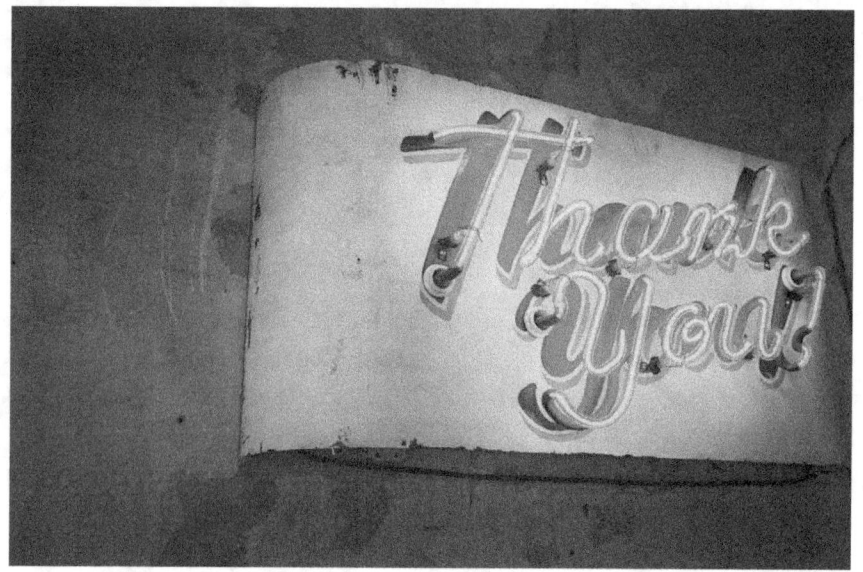